Unthinkable:
Tips for Surviving a Child's
Traumatic Brain Injury

> **A CAREGIVER'S COMPANION**

Dixie Fremont-Smith Coskie

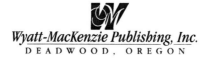

Wyatt-MacKenzie Publishing, Inc.
DEADWOOD, OREGON

DISCLAIMER

*The information contained in this book
should not be taken as medical advice.*

Unthinkable:
Tips for Surviving a Child's
Traumatic Brain Injury

by Dixie Fremont-Smith Coskie

ISBN: 978-1-936214-41-9

©2011 Dixie Fremont-Smith Coskie

Excerpt from *Unthinkable: A Mother's Tragedy, Terror, and Triumph
through a Child's Traumatic Brain Injury*

www.DixieCoskie.com

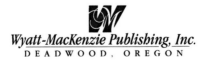

Wyatt-MacKenzie Publishing, Inc.
DEADWOOD, OREGON

15115 Highway 36, Deadwood, Oregon 97430
541-964-3314 ⋆ www.wyattmackenzie.com

Dedicated to the entire Coskie family.

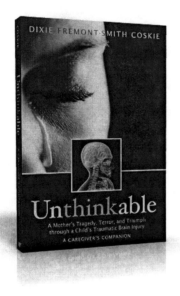

Unthinkable: A Mother's Tragedy, Terror, and Triumph through a Child's Traumatic Brain Injury is written from a mother's perspective. It's an account of surviving tragedy is filled with universal lessons about struggle and triumph. It will bring you into a realm where body, mind and spirit are pushed to their limits. It shares a personal experience and a mother's heart and knowledge. *Unthinkable* offers hope where no hope seems possible.

Unthinkable is different; its raw emotion is honest and thought-provoking, with the essential uplifting elements of belief, strength and perseverance. Dixie writes of her internal struggles to find meaning in her son's pain, as she comes to find the simplest of things important—when her son is able to blink his eyelids again, lift his finger, utter a word.

Available on Amazon.com in Paperback and Kindle

Introduction

We had the privilege of publishing Dixie's book *Unthinkable: A Mother's Tragedy, Terror, and Triumph through a Child's Traumatic Brain Injury* in 2010. We received so many requests for the valuable tips which ran after Dixie's chapters to be packaged in a format all their own—here they are.

May you and your family never be in need of these trauma tips, but may knowing them give you the wisdom Dixie drew from the unthinkable trauma her son suffered.

~ Wyatt-MacKenzie Publishing

Everyone in life at some point or another will have
  to face grief, suffering, and death
The only thing you have power over is how you will
  react to life—or possibly death
Fairytale endings do not always play out in real life

~ Dixie

TABLE OF CONTENTS

7 Acceptance

8 Transitioning

9 Going Forward

10 Siblings

Afterword

1

Be Prepared

Be Prepared Before an Accident Happens

- Have a "values" history—a statement of personal values regarding your health care wishes in the event of a life-threatening illness or accident. For example, would you want to be resuscitated or not?

- Have a living will, ie, a simple statement regarding your wishes on whether you want heroic medical care or measures to be taken or not if you become terminally ill.

- Choose a proxy. Designate a person who will make life-or-death decisions for you in case of emergency or if you cannot speak for yourself for any reason (also known as a durable power of attorney for a health care proxy).

- Discuss and have in writing the wishes of all family members regarding whether they would want to be an organ donor.

- Make a will and keep it up-to-date.

- Keep two stocked emergency kits, one in your kitchen and one in your car. An ideal first-aid kit should include the following materials:

  ◦ A first-aid book

  ◦ Bandaging materials, including band-aids, antiseptic solution, alcohol pads, soap or other cleansing agent, a lubricant (eg, petroleum jelly), sterile adhesive bandages in different sizes, nonstick sterile pads, cotton rolls, instant cold compresses, a pair of metal scissors, and sterile rubber gloves (2 pairs)

   ◦ A thermometer and a warm blanket

   ◦ Medications, both nonprescription drugs (eg, aspirin, acetamino-
     phen for pain relief) and, if possible, certain prescription drugs (eg,
     insulin or an asthma inhaler)

   ◦ A flash light and radio, both with extra batteries

• Keep lists of all emergency numbers handy: police, fire, poison control,
  doctors, hospitals, lawyers; also keep your health insurance and social
  security numbers and cards handy.

• Make sure the following phone numbers are in the contact list of your
  home and cell phones: family members, neighbors, doctor's office,
  drug store, school contacts.

• Carry a cell phone, and make it a habit to keep it charged.

• Keep a list of all medications that any of your children are currently
  taking written down in a convenient place, such as your wallet.

• Keep physicals of all family members up to date.

• Keep medical records of all family members in a safe and convenient
  place.

2

Traumatic Event

At the Accident Scene

• Do not panic

• Assess the situation and bodily injuries, but do not move the body.

• Ask if anyone knows CPR or if there is a doctor present.

• Put pressure on any severely bleeding wounds.

• Ask someone to call 911 and your spouse/partner.

• Keep the victim warm (ask if anyone has a blanket, use jackets, etc).

• Ask someone to direct traffic until police arrive.

• Let the police deal with traffic control, the witnesses, and the details of what happened.

• Breathe in and out; wait for the ambulance; pray.

• If you are not allowed in the ambulance, ask a neighbor or friend to drive you to the emergency room.

In the Emergency Room

• Although you will be severely stressed, before signing forms for any procedure to be done, ASK what you are signing and what the consequences will be for doing so, as well as what the consequences will be if you do not. For example, what are the risks and potential complications? What kind of burdens and side effects will the proposed treatment impose?

• Stay out of the way so the medical personnel can do what's needed, but don't leave your child unless the doctors insist or you are feeling queasy, faint, or about to throw up. If you feel ill, let a nurse know.

• Ask questions when appropriate. What's going on? How extensive are the injuries? Are the injuries life-threatening? What is being done?

• Do not become hysterical; losing control will promptly land you in the waiting area, away from your child.

• If the injuries are life-threatening and you are religious, ask for a chaplain, priest, rabbi, or spiritual director.

• If your child is taken to a trauma center, ask if you accompany him or her in the ambulance or helicopter. If not, have a friend or neighbor drive you to the trauma center. Do not drive yourself.

In the Trauma Center

• Find out who is in charge.

• Ask for updates from the nurses and doctors.

• Stay in the room or area where medical personnel ask you to so that they can find you right away.

• Ask if you can see your child.

• Find out what tests have been done, are being done, will be done and why. If you don't understand the answers, ask again—and again, until you do.

• Ask doctors to explain terms such as closed or open head injury or fracture, shearing of the brain, internal hemorrhage, intracranial pressure, blood clot, seizures, neurosurgeon, MRI, CT scan, EEG, post-traumatic amnesia, retrograde amnesia, anterograde amnesia, coma, etc.

- Know that brain injury is usually described as mild, moderate, or severe. The length of time that a person is in a coma is one of the many factors that can determine the severity of an injury.

- Certain tests, such as the Glasgow Coma Scale, help medical staff evaluate level of consciousness. The Rancho Los Amigos scale is a more detailed test that describes the behaviors and abilities of a person who is gradually coming out a coma.

- Ask your doctor if the Glasgow or Rancho scale has been used to evaluate your child. Ask him or her to explain what the numbers mean and if there has been any change since the injury. Ask what may happen next.

- Know that the length of coma varies for each person, because every brain injury is different. Your child will not just suddenly awaken; it is a slow, painstaking process.

- Seeing your child unconscious for the first time will undoubtedly be an emotional shock.

- Ask if your child has other injuries, such as broken bones, internal injuries, etc.

- Decide on one family member or friend who can act as the contact person for other family members and friends. Relay forthcoming medical information to the contact person, and give him or her the authority to give updates to others.

- Have your contact person compile a list of family members and neighbors who would like to receive continuing information, and ask him or her to phone or e-mail updates when any new information becomes available.

- Ask for pen and paper to start chronicling the names of doctors and nurses, procedures, medications, and any medical questions that arise.

- Recognize that the possible effects after brain injury include not only medical and physical changes, but also changes in cognition, communication, behavior, and even personality.

• Appreciate that each child's situation, symptoms, and recovery are unique.

In the ICU

• Be patient; pray if praying is a part of your belief system.

• Don't be ashamed to cry or to ask more and more questions.

• Talk to your child, hold his or her hand, and believe that he or she can hear you. Ask him or her to please give you a sign that he or she can hear you. Let your child know you are there and that you will not leave him or her. Reassure your child that he or she is receiving good care.

• Get to know the surroundings. Ask about the equipment and monitors in the room, such as how to read information such as heart rate, pulse, and oxygen levels. Ask a nurse to explain the purpose of each tube. Ask how to operate the hospital bed.

• Ask for the names, purposes, and possible side effects of all medications that are being administered. Ask about the time intervals of dosages. Write down this information as well as any procedures being done and any questions you have.

• Find the locations of the light switches, the coffee machine, the time-out areas, the bathroom and waiting area for visitors, and cots for parents.

• Find a private area in the hospital where you can meet your spouse or significant other to talk and cry in private.

• Ask and demand that you can spend the days and nights with your child.

• Get to know the nurses; you'll soon learn which ones are the most helpful and which ones are less so.

• When any medication is being administered, check and double-check the name of the drug and the dosage.

• Realize that nurses work in shifts and are not "on" every day. They could not possibly always be up-to-date with changes being made in procedures or with all medication changes; you need to be aware to watch and help if you can.

• Seek out a social worker. He or she can help during this tremendously emotional time and can also help you with your insurance company to retain a case worker to follow your medical case and work with you on financial coverage.

• If your child is about to turn eighteen, many states require that families notify the insurance carrier of the child's disability for the health insurance to continue under the family's plan.

• Government programs such as Medicaid and/or Medicare may help with medical costs.

• The department of insurance in your state may help with problems such as being uninsured or underinsured.

• If your child is eighteen or older, he or she is a legal adult and has the power to make all medical decisions. If your child is impaired and not able to make decisions, you may consider becoming his or her legal guardian.

• Allow yourself time to feel what you are feeling and to express those feelings. Anger, extreme sadness, and grief are normal.

• If you have not been very religious in the past, perhaps you will feel your spiritual life awakening or past religious beliefs surfacing.

• Call your employer, let them know the situation and that you will not be coming to work.

• Take time to bring other family members up to date; regularly call your contact person to relay information.

• Make sure you have put someone you trust in charge of taking care of your other children so that you and your spouse/partner can focus on your injured child.

• If you are not married or don't have a good relationship with your spouse/partner, ask a friend to stay with you at the ICU.

• Search for hope; ask to talk to a social worker or spiritual director, or seek out other parents who have gone through a severe head injury in a child. Learn of their experience…and their recovery.

• Be awake and ready to talk to doctors early in the morning when they make their rounds. Have your questions ready. For example, is my child stable? Responding to the medications? What can we expect? When—or will—he or she awaken? What can we do?

• Trust the nurses when they ask you to take a walk, go to the café, get some sleep, go home, take a nap, talk to your spouse. Be patient.

• Don't try to project what will happen in the next two weeks or two years—live and deal in the moment.

• Set a schedule. Try to have one parent home for your other kids, and one at the hospital for the injured child. If you are divorced, try to put differences aside. If one parent is not available, enlist another family member or friend.

• Don't forget about your other children at home. Check on them by phone, text messaging or e-mail. Reassure them and allow them to cry, vent, and show their fears. Try to best answer their questions, and when words cannot console…pray.

• Seek out someone other than your spouse/partner to express your fears and frustrations. Find someone who will listen and not judge.

• Try to understand the situation is not caused by you or God—get rid of guilt.

• Know the difference between coma, induced coma, and persistent vegetative state.

• Consult the ethics personnel at the hospital so that you become informed on how the hospital deals with issues such as continuing life supports or allowing one to die.

• Continue to ask questions and know everyone involved in your child's treatment; this will include numerous health care personnel, including the ICU personnel, trauma doctors, neurosurgeons, plastic surgeons, respiratory nurses, physical therapists, occupational therapists, speech therapists, social workers, financial advisors, and more.

• Realize that your emotions, which are likely to be many, strong, and swing frequently, are normal: anger, denial, forgetfulness, disorganization, confusion, feeling disconnected and alone.

• Having arguments and disagreements with your spouse/partner is normal; you are both under tremendous stress.

• Forgive quickly and move on so as not to add even more stress to the situation.

• Vent your anger alone, perhaps while driving to and from the hospital, or just have time to cry in private.

• Think and visualize positive thoughts. Be conscious of your breathing and think positive in any way you can.

Advocate for Your Child

• Make sure your child receives his or her medications and is treated with dignity. This includes having appropriate undergarments; having catheters, IV lines, or diapers changed in a reasonable timeframe; and having daily sponge baths.

• Always discuss pressing issues outside of your child's room; always try to instill hope in your child's presence, as if he or she can hear you (and maybe he or she can).

• Know that your child's response to pain, though heartbreaking, can be a positive sign.

• Try not to get involved with other families' or patients' drama in the ICU.

• Know key words such as tracheotomy, ventilator, respirator, skull fractures, contusions, concussion, *storming*, etc.

- Educate yourself on brain injury and related medical issues. Ask for books, magazines…anything that will help you better understand words such as acnosia, agraphia, anomia, anosmia, alexia, ambulate, etc.

- Understand that a brain injury can ultimately cause problems with how a person moves, thinks, communicates, feels, and behaves.

- Know that you cannot give what you do not have.

- Know your limits and what you can and cannot do. For example, can I watch a bloody procedure? Can I stay here one more night?

- It's normal for siblings to have conflict; they may resist going to school or studying, or act out. Let teachers know what happened and seek out school counselors to help with the new terrain, because your priority at this time must be with your injured child.

- Keep up to date with your child's medical issues—talk hourly with the doctors and nurses—and never stop talking and asking questions.

- Never stop talking to your child and reassuring him or her that he or she is going to get better. No one knows for certain if people in comas can hear, so it's best to assume they can and act accordingly.

- Know who the doctor is who is ultimately in charge of your child's case. This doctor is your child's health care team leader. Like nurses, doctors work different shifts, and the specific doctor who looked at your child today may not be back for several more days.

- If you have any problems or personality conflicts with any nurse, let the head nurse know the problem.

- If you have any problems with a particular doctor, consult with the ICU supervisor.

Preparing Your Other Children and Grandparents for a Visit to the ICU

• Ask friends and acquaintances to not visit the ICU at this crucial time; let them know they are important to you and that you will need them later in recovery.

• Call home daily to give age-appropriate answers to your children's questions, but do not get caught in details.

• Help children understand why and how the injury happened. Younger children often blame themselves for the incident, while older children may question if they could have prevented the injury; reassure them there was nothing they could have done.

• Give reassurance that the injured child is getting good care.

• When you feel the need to bring your other children to the hospital, talk to the hospital's child life department, which helps siblings and grandparents cope with the situation and prepare for their visit.

• Never force your other children to visit; wait for them to ask, and wait until they are ready to arrange the visit. Help prepare children by giving them age-appropriate written and verbal information on brain injury. Give them time to absorb the information and the situation.

• Encourage your other children to write cards or send pictures to help decorate the hospital room.

• If siblings have become "quiet," do not assume that they are okay or have accepted the situation; often, they do not want to add to your burden.

• Have someone else bring your other children to the hospital to visit their brother or sister. Make sure you have described the situation to prepare them; show them a picture of the injured child lying in bed, surrounded by the machines, and try to explain how the monitors and doctors are helping.

• Be truthful. Explain what the doctors are doing and hope to accomplish, but also let children (in age-appropriate terms) and grandparents know the reality of life and possible death. Ask everyone to trust in God.

• Give children and grandparents permission to cry and to talk about their feelings.

What Friends Can Do

• Ask a friend to pack and bring a small suitcase for the parents to the ICU: toiletries, change of clothes, sweats, sweatshirts, comfortable t-shirts, small blanket, small medical dictionary, important phone numbers and e-mail addresses, pocket book, camera, gum, small snacks, a blank notebook and pen, a copy of this book.

• Listen, be patient, give hope.

• If you are new to your community and do not know many people, contact your nearest neighbors, local organizations, or your church for assistance,

• Ask a good friend to take charge of scheduling other friends and neighbors to help with cleaning, yard work, childcare, carpooling, and grocery shopping.

• Organize a food schedule with kid-friendly meals for the other children. Tell the cooks of any allergies the children may have. Keep all containers disposable. Set a consistent time of day to drop off the meals. Paper cups, towels, and plates are helpful.

• Buy gift cards: coffee, gas, fast food, and for any restaurants near the hospital.

• Put together an e-mail and phone list to keep others up to date.

• Think about organizing a fundraiser for the future.

• Hold on to hope.

• Pray.

What Friends Should Not Do

• Don't try to avoid the parents, but give them their space when needed.

• Don't offer advice, pity phrases, or quick solutions, such as "I know what you're going through," "You should _____," "Time heals all wounds," or "You'll be okay."

• Don't pry into personal matters, but be there to listen whenever your friend wants to talk or tell you something.

3

Rehabilitation

Getting Ready for the Transition to a
Rehabilitation Hospital

• The ICU's job is to stabilize the patient. Understand that when your child is stable, you will need to investigate the option of taking him or her to a rehabilitation hospital.

• Have another family member at the ICU to advocate for your child while you're investigating potential rehabilitation hospitals.

• Talk to a social worker about the transition ahead.

• Find out what do rehabilitation hospitals actually do. Rehabilitation is to assist your child in regaining or gaining maximal independence. Rehabilitation helps the survivor to relearn old skills, acquire new skills, and develop skills that have been lost or that will not develop.

• Know that rehabilitation requires a comprehensive team approach. The family's involvement is crucial.

• Depending on the severity and location of your child's brain injury, recognize that the outcome of therapy may differ.

• Learn some basic brain physiology. Neurons are cells in the brain that send messages to other parts of the brain and body. Damage to these neurons can be temporary, and they may recover on their own. Damage can also be permanent, which could result in the loss of certain abilities. In some cases, other neurons make new connections and take over the job of the damaged neurons.

Visiting a Potential Rehabilitation Hospital

• Understand the duration of your stay at the rehabilitation hospital is likely to be unsure. Your child could be there 3 weeks, 3 months, or 3 years.

• Take into account the distance from your home to the rehab hospital, as well as parking and traffic issues. For example, will you have to pay for parking?

• Realize the doctors and nurses you are currently working with in the ICU will no longer follow your case or have any input.

• Recognize that facilities differ; not all can manage someone on a ventilator or with a tracheotomy, or care for an individual with behavioral issues. Some facilities have different types of care for someone who is in a coma or catatonic versus someone who is more independent.

• Tour different facilities and watch therapies in action.

• Ask to speak to former patients and/or their caregivers about their experience at the facility.

• When visiting the facility, bring your spouse/partner or another family member or friend with you.

• Take notes or bring a voice recording device. Be prepared with questions.

First Impressions Are Often Right

• Pay attention to how you feel when you first walk in.

• Note if the people appear friendly and professional.

• Are you seen in a reasonable amount of time?

• Do the premises appear to be well maintained, clean, safe, etc?

• Were all your questions answered?

• Was the staff compassionate?

Questions to Ask

• What will be the source of funding?

• How is this facility accredited?

• Is there a waiting list?

• Is there a head doctor on the floor at all times?

• What is the nurse-to-patient ratio?

• What is the turnover of staff?

• Is there bilingual staff?

• How often will my child receive services? How long are the sessions?

• What is your success rate for patients with traumatic brain injuries?

• Can I speak to other patients who have been here?

• What therapies are offered?

• Do you have a special brace clinic or orthopedics department?

• Do you have a therapeutic aquatics department?

• What about assistive technology?

• Do you provide tutors for school work?

• Do you have counselors or social workers? Do you provide family therapy?

• Can my other children visit? What is the involvement of family?

• Can I sleep in the room and be with my child twenty-four hours a day?

• Is there a chapel, cafeteria, separate bathrooms, or sleeping areas for parents?

• What are my rights?

• Do you help with the transition home?

Making the Transition from the Rehabilitation Hospital

• It's okay to feel apprehensive as you leave the ICU.

• Communicate feelings with your spouse/partner; try to comfort each other.

• Be prepared that the atmosphere in the rehabilitation hospital will be more subdued than in the ICU.

• Find out where the resource room or library is and where you can get Internet access to learn more about traumatic brain injury.

• Be prepared to see very disabled children, wheelchairs, walkers, etc.

• Understand medical terminology such as catatonic, vegetative state, etc.

• Know that your child may need to share a room with another patient; ask for a patient in the same age range and sex of your child.

• Have one parent stay in the hospital, while the other is at home with the other children.

• Set a time of day when you can connect with your spouse/partner by phone or e-mail.

• Bring in items from home: I-pod, radio, clothes, posters, pictures, diary, pillows, etc.

• Call home to talk to your other children; answer their questions as best you can according to their age level of understanding.

• Rest when you can.

• Get ready to fight the fight of your life.

• Write down the names of all therapies and the names of all therapists, nurses, and doctors.

• Know the names of the medications your child is now on and when they need to be administered. Advocate for your child when the nurses are late in administering drugs or changing the bed or undergarments.

• Ask where the cafeteria is. Are coupons provided for parking or meals?

• Talk to a financial advisor at the hospital and find out about resources they provide.

• Talk with a social worker about getting a case worker involved from your insurance company.

• Stay with your child or have another adult at the rehab hospital twenty-four hours a day.

• You may begin to realize that there might be long-term effects from the injury and begin to feel intense fear and anxiety.

• You may face the loss of what might have been.

4

Returning

Returning to Work

- Make a realistic plan with your employer as to when to come back to work, possibly working part-time or from the hospital or home. For some, returning to work is a welcome change. It can create a break from what has been an ever-present grief. The office may be the only part of life that seems normal and routine. But for many who have experienced a recent loss or a traumatic experience, returning to work can be difficult. You may be dreading the thought of returning to work for several reasons:

- Not being at the hospital to help your injured child, or at home to help your spouse/partner and other children.

- Seeing coworkers for the first time exposes you to "I'm so sorry" comments, which continually reminds you of your situation. A gentle "thank you" is all the response that is necessary. You do not need to give any more information you do not wish to share.

- You may have a high-pressure job with many deadlines and little room for mistakes. You have probably noticed that it is difficult to concentrate and retain information in your grief. You may be easily distracted, and errors can occur. It is useful to check everything twice, or to ask a coworker or supervisor to review what you have done. If you choose, share with your coworkers or supervisors how difficult things seem at this time and when you need their help or space.

- You may worry about breaking down in front of colleagues or in the middle of an important meeting. This can happen, but save yourself embarrassment by briefly letting people know what has occurred in your life. If you need to excuse yourself, do so. Take as much time off as allowed and then some to regain control and some sort of stability… take small steps…it is "one day at a time."

There is No Right or Wrong Way to Grieve

• Grief often comes in waves.

• Denial: "This can't be happening to me."

• Anger: "Why is this happening? Who is to blame?"

• Bargaining: "Make this not happen, and I in turn will _____."

• Depression: "I am too sad to do anything, physically, emotionally, mentally, spiritually."

• Acceptance: "I am at peace with what has happened and is going to happen."

5

Expectations

Rehabilitation: What to Expect, What to Do, What to Say

• Be patient, the healing process is slow.

• Be prepared to be lonely, very lonely. Life as you once knew it has changed…forever. Invite your friends to visit for short times.

• Invite friends of the injured child. Prepare them ahead of time, and keep their visits short. Stay in the room with them.

• Have family members give you a break and stay with your child while you sleep, nap, take a walk, or when you need to connect with your partner.

• Seek out positive people to give you hope: counselors, clergy, friends, a special nurse.

• Recognize that all of the following can be symptoms of grief: changes in appetite or weight, sleep disturbances, exhaustion, the desire to withdraw or run away, numbness, anxiety, argumentativeness, hopelessness.

• Know and accept that you cannot give what you do not have. Allow your emotions to surface to work through them.

• Your family may be suffering other losses: familiar routines, sense of identity and security, feeling of being in control of life situations, income, carefree days, and the normalcy of everyday life.

- If you are estranged from your faith community or have none, consider reconnecting or exploring alternatives.

- Consider joining a support group for people dealing with traumatic brain injury.

- Remember that grief is a natural response to loss; it does not have to be a way of life.

- Don't give up on your child, God, doctors, therapists, your spouse/ partner, or yourself.

- Depending on the cause of your child's traumatic brain injury, you may want to look into legal counsel. Brain injury claims are complex and can cause further hardship to your family. It is important to hire a lawyer who has experience in brain injury cases.

- Be aware that your other children may fall behind in school, act out, or become depressed.

- Seek help through the school or the hospital's counseling department.

- When you are home with your other children, concentrate on helping them. When you are at the rehabilitation hospital, try to concentrate only on your injured child.

- Realize that life goes on for the rest of the world while you are trying to adjust to your new situation.

- Try to keep abreast of the news in the world.

- Pray for others.

- Don't start drinking alcohol or doing drugs to escape your reality.

- Talk to the speech, occupational, and physical therapists before or after each session. Ask questions. Know the goals of therapy and your child's limitations. Ask if you can participate with therapies, but also learn when to back off.

- Never stop talking and reassuring your child that you are near and promising him or her that he or she is going to get better.

- Be committed to your child's success.

- Keep fighting.

- Get to know the nurses.

- Seek counseling together with your spouse/partner if issues and discrepancies arise, or if you find that you are distancing yourself from one another.

- It's understandable that your sex life will dwindle or become nonexistent.

- Realize that your friends and family do not understand what you are going through, and you should not feel pressure to explain it.

- Let family members know you do not have any more energy to extend their way to help them with their grief; ask them to seek the comfort of other family members.

- As the bills, and more and more bills, arrive, ask your case worker for help with the insurance and to help you seek medical assistance, including Medicaid, state health funding, government grants, etc.

- The primary breadwinner of the family needs to stay productive to maintain health insurance, a job, a pay check, etc.

- Be patient with others as they may complain of their problems, which seem trivial in comparison with yours. Remember everyone's pain is his or her own.

- Continue writing into your own personal diary. Take pictures or video-tape the process of progress and improvement.

- Trying to take care of your other children's emotions when they visit the rehabilitation hospital can be challenging. Do it in shifts and try to have a nurse, friend, or your spouse/ partner with you.

- When you are at home, find time to talk to each child alone and on his or her level. For example, take one child with you while you run errands, or for a special ice cream treat and a talk.

• Meet as a family to find out how everyone is coping.

• Be generous with hugs.

• Ask your children to help by cleaning up after themselves, taking care of each other, being more independent with homework, etc. Let them know that counseling and a support system are there when they are ready.

• Educate yourself further on traumatic brain injury and the recovery process.

• Listen, stay alert to all the information you are trying to process.

• Try not to think or dwell on the other patients in the hospital.

• Remember: patience, fortitude, and perseverance can transform your life.

• If your child cannot talk, use blinking response or "thumbs-up" tactics.

• Play popular music that your child likes.

• As exhaustion sets in, try to sleep when you can or talk to your doctor about medication.

• Know that your moods and those of your other children will change daily when critical moments and difficult situations arise.

• Recognize that your other children have suddenly been thrown into adult issues and adult stresses. It's normal for older sons and daughters to compensate by doing things that a parent used to do, such as taking over household chores or disciplining younger children, in an effort to try to take control of something...

• Because it is impossible to personally thank everyone in your community for all their help, put a short thank-you blurb into your local newspaper. If you don't have the strength, ask someone to write it for you.

6

Self-Care

Self-Care for Caregivers

- Take care of yourself. Eat three meals a day and drink plenty of water.

- Realize you are not alone; other people before you have experienced your sorrow and have potentially come through the tunnel.

- Don't worry too much about how other extended family members are coping. Concentrate on your child, yourself, your other children, and your spouse/partner.

- Questions like "Why you? Why me? Why did this happen?" are normal and may never be resolved.

- Know that nothing you could have said or did could have changed the circumstances.

- Have weekly team meetings with doctors and therapists.

- Celebrate small gains.

- Know that every head injury is different and that predicting future gains or future setbacks might be impossible.

- If possible, take your child outside to feel the fresh air.

- Be patient. Pray.

- Enlist help to help you juggle work, home life, and the hospital routine. Coworkers, older children, and friends can relieve you of some responsibilities and even give you a break at the hospital.

- Check in with your children's school counselors and teachers often. Siblings often hide their feelings. Be on the lookout for changes in behavior in your other children, such as frequent sadness, crying, hopelessness, feelings of worthlessness, guilt, apathy, low energy, loss of interest in activities that used to be enjoyable, difficulty concentrating or making decisions, major changes in sleeping or eating habits, increased anger or irritability, thinking or talking about suicide or death. Depending on the signs and symptoms, your other children may need psychiatric evaluations or antidepressants.

- Every minute you have, try to stimulate your child's brain.

- Live in the moment. Let life slow down. Hope.

- Rest.

- If your child responds more to one person, ask him or her to visit more often.

- Take time to connect with your spouse/partner outside the hospital and your home. Meet for a quick lunch or take a walk together. Let your spouse/partner know that he or she is loved. Try to find something to laugh about.

- Every day, know that a little more pain and a little bit more struggle can regain a little more movement.

- Although the holidays will never be like they used to, try to make them as normal as possible by keeping with your traditions. Ask a friend to shop and decorate for you.

- When you are not home, designate a neighbor or friend to be called in case of an emergency.

- Plan your driving route to and from the rehab hospital before or after the morning rush and before the evening rush hour traffic.

- The games and therapies the occupational and physical therapists use may seem childlike, but they will progress as your child makes gains.

- If you become the target of your child's anger, resist the urge to blame yourself. You will not be able to erase what has happened.

• As hard as it is, try to take time away from the hospital to give attention to your other children.

• Celebrate milestones: first time speaking, moving a finger, making eye contact…

• Help continue therapies at night when the therapists leave. Know the routine and what you can be doing, such as massaging limbs, reading books, reciting the A, B, C's, playing cards, etc.

• When it is time for toilet re-training for your child, ask for a nurse of the same sex to help.

• Realize that when your child is looking at you, he or she may not be able to recognize or remember you, or process who you are.

• Don't be startled or alarmed if your child show signs of anger or has other behavior changes.

• If you have personality conflicts with any psychiatrists, doctors, or nurses, let your case manager know; he or she will help ease the tension.

• Try not to feel frustrated about the many things that are out of your control. Some examples include feeling that your expectations have not been met if your child's progress slows down and seems to stop, becoming angry at the hospital or rehabilitation staff because you feel that they are not doing everything they can to make your child better, feeling that your child is not trying hard enough, feeling angry at your child for putting you into this situation, and seeing small gains and little improvement after working so hard and putting your life on hold.

• Accept the realization that recovery may be lifelong.

• Know the possible realities of permanent loss of memory, mobility, hearing, sight, or speech.

• Accept the possibility that the person you knew may never be returned to you.

• Remember your child is alive!

• Be thankful for committed therapists; you're moving forward.

• Remember that small gains are big miracles.

• Take a needed break away from the stress of caring for your injured child and your other children. Nurture your relationship with your spouse/partner—have sex! Go to a nearby hotel, cry and talk and rekindle your relationship.

• Know that your child will be okay if you leave. Take time out on a day when a trusted family member and a special nurse can be there.

• Come out of your own suffering to possibly help a new patient or family just beginning this journey.

• Remember that the monotony of the days could be worse; your child could be dead or not progressing.

• When sharing a hospital room with another patient and his or her parents, remain tactful and patient. Keep a sense of humor. Repeat to yourself "This too shall pass."

• Although you cannot understand the daily trials mixed with your joys and sorrows, try to believe that God knows all and He has a divine plan.

• Keep a separate journal in the hospital room to share with your spouse/partner updates of progress from therapies during the day. Inform each other what has happened, including doctor's conversations and any changes in medication.

• After your child has gone to bed and you know your other children are asleep, call home and connect with your spouse/partner.

• Go to bed with thanksgiving and praise and ready to begin the fight the next day!

7

Acceptance

Preparing for the First Visit Home

- The first visit home is equally terrifying and filled with happiness.

- Your visit home will be full of trial and error and will give you great insight into how hard it will be when your child finally returns home permanently—the caregiving and caregiving and caregiving.

- Be prepared for reactions from your injured child as well as from your other children. They will be apprehensive and unsure as to how life could ever be the same. Be reassuring; you all will slowly adjust to the changes with time and with help from each other.

- Know that a lot of emotions will surface when your child has to return to the hospital at the end of the day.

- Memory issues are a huge problem for victims of traumatic brain injury, and they affect the whole family. Using a whiteboard and calendar can help if your child is able to read. Reinforce the day's schedule, what activities were accomplished, what is happening next, etc.

- If your child lashes out in anger, talk softly and in a reassuring voice. If the anger persists, walk away until your child has time to calm down.

- Remind yourself of the progress your child is making and believe that he or she will heal.

- Keep fighting! Your child is a miracle in progress.

- Keep advocating for the needs of your family and the needs of your child, especially around the holidays.

• Get a journal for your child's therapist to record daily goals. This lets your child know what is expected and reassures your child that he or she is accomplishing a lot.

• Put pictures of the therapists in the journal so your child can remember their faces and names.

• Give thanks for visits home and time together as a family.

• Begin the plan for the transition home. Start talking with doctors and counselors. Take advantage of your safety net while you can because soon you will be on your own.

• Remain hopeful.

• Your child has come a long way, but the reality is that he or she still has a long way to go.

• Your child may continue to be dealing with both physical and mental issues, including mobility, memory, speech, and self-care, and is unlikely to be fully independent.

• Therapy services may be coming to an end, and you may be dealing with insurance issues. Doctors and therapists may recommend that you start planning for the transition back to your home, including possibly looking into outpatient therapies or a special needs programs, or possibly a boarding school to fulfill all of your child's needs. Ask for references and recommendations of schools and rehabilitation hospitals in your area and start to visit and begin the interviewing process. You may also want to consider facilities beyond your local area if they specialize in your child's specific needs.

• Bringing your child home or taking him or her to another facility is one of the hardest decisions you will have to make. There is no right or wrong answer, although taking him or her to a nursing home that does not offer occupational, physical, or speech therapies may mean little further gain in the recovery process.

• Caregiving is never ending and exhausting. Recognize your own limitations and what you can and cannot do.

8

Transitioning

Transitioning Home

- Before you leave the rehabilitation hospital, apply through the bureau of motor vehicles in your state for a handicapped placard or plate. The rehabilitation hospital may have the paperwork, and all you have to do is sign and mail.

- Have all assistive equipment ready to go: car/van, handicapped ramp, wheelchair, bed, bathrooms renovated for handicap accessibility.

- Set up home care with the traveling nurse's organization. The rehabilitation hospital can guide you through this.

- Your family's life will probably never be as it was before. For a time be prepared for meals uncooked, laundry undone, and the cares of your other children to be placed on a back burner. Your marriage will remain on hold for awhile or at least function in a different way. If you can afford it, hire a housekeeper, nanny, marriage counselor, etc, if needed.

- Never stop trying to stimulate your child's mind: How much is 2+2? What color is this? Play a board game, do a puzzle, name the planets or types of trees, talk about cities or countries, etc.

- Caregiving requires not only a lot of patience and stamina but also understanding. Know what you're up against: Can you leave your child alone for a moment? Does your child understand the stove is on? Can you keep track of all the medications and maintenance of wheelchairs, walkers, braces, etc?

- If you choose to bring your child home, do not do so for selfish reasons: a professional facility may be better prepared to initially help in your child's healing process, and your child could return home at a later date. Look at all options! Consider what will be best for your child and the rest of your family; after you make your decision, move forward, be determined to help in the healing process, and never look back.

• Talk with administrators, doctors, therapists, teachers, family, and insurance companies…you must advocate for your child!

• Prepare your other kids for changes ahead. They may feel embarrassed by the behaviors of the injured child and may avoid being home or inviting friends over.

• Some children may think their brother or sister is cured when it's time to return home. Let them know injuries still linger and what they are: cognitive, physical…

• The therapist will do a home assessment and let you know how you can plan for your child's return home: wheelchair ramp-guard rails, special utensils, a handicapped bed and bathrooms…

• You may begin to start to think of reality and wonder how you are going to cope with all the new changes and challenges, physically, financially, and emotionally. Vent your concerns to someone who can help and direct you. Social worker, case worker, doctor…friend.

• You have been at the rehabilitation hospital for so long you may feel desperate to leave, but be patient until everything is ready for your child's arrival home.

• Give thanks for huge miracles—your child is moving on…thank all the therapists and doctors. Perhaps give them a card with a picture of them and your child…ask a friend to bake cookies for the nurses…

• The joy of being home may be fleeting as you realize all the challenges ahead.

• Others in your community may think that just because you are home you may no longer need help. Communicate that you are still in need of help! Cooking, cleaning, childcare, carpools…and comfort.

• Your family will go through many adjustments. Don't give up—it's trial and error.

- Your child's limitations may be more prevalent; now you will become your child's nutritionist, chauffeur, self-care person, as well as occupational, physical, and speech therapists! Put into practice all that you have learned over these long and hard months.

- Search out resources to help…and keep in touch with doctors and therapists from your rehabilitation hospital. Know too that they soon will not be involved in treatment and that you will move on…with outpatient therapies or with another facility.

At Home

- You have been absent from home for weeks or months and sometimes years, and your other children probably have felt abandoned; they may resent you suddenly being home and taking over again and instilling new demands. Your whole family will go through a transition period, readjusting to a new way of life, trying to find some sort of a "new" normalcy.

- Give thanks.

- Set up a consistent daily schedule.

- Implement a home therapy program: speech therapy, occupational therapy, physical therapy.

- Start investigating outpatient facilities or start therapies.

- Start planning the transition back to school.

- Know your child's limitations.

- Suggest ways in which your other children can help, or give them permission to back off.

- Invite friends over in small numbers and for short times.

- Refill medications as needed.

- Be patient with yourself and others as you all adjust to the changes.

- Schedule in-home nursing staff as medically needed.

Transitioning to an Outpatient Facility

• Be prepared for a lot of driving back and forth to and from the facility; stimulate your child's mind in the car…review multiplication tables, play games such as On My Way To My Grandmother's House…

• Enlist others to help drive to and from the facility. Perhaps you may qualify for state-funded transportation.

• You may find that the injuries of other patients in the new facility are not as severe as those in the rehabilitation hospital: broken legs, hip replacements, surgical recovery.

• You may be thrown into a more adult atmosphere if the facility is not pediatric in nature.

• Everyone there is seeking some sort of relief, wanting to regain dignity, self-worth, and pride in his or her life.

• Remember that how you react to any given situation is in your power.

• You will have to adjust to other's reactions when they see your child in public. Smile, be polite, and say a prayer that they will never have to be in your position.

• You may want to invite a small gathering of your child's friends over to the house so they all can get reacquainted before or if your child returns to school.

• You may wonder how your child will be accepted back into the circle of his or her peers. It will be an adjustment for everyone, and only time will tell.

• You may be feeling isolated, frustrated by comments about being over-protective, unable to think about the future.

• Outpatient therapy is very different from inpatient therapy; it feels more like a business, getting a patient in and out every half hour without much personal interaction.

• You may be worried about the new staff or uncertain as to what to expect during this next phase of recovery in outpatient therapy.

• The exercises are relentless; continue with an at-home regimen.

- Be thankful that your child is at this stage and is still progressing; many survivors of traumatic brain injury plateau early and do not progress to higher functioning levels, leaving a life that is not "productive" and a shattered family.

- Be thankful that your family is all together under one roof.

Transitioning Back to School

- Usually, brain healing shows the most progress in the first year after the traumatic injury. It is crucial to stimulate the brain properly with strategies known to help survivors to succeed.

- Some school systems need help and guidance from parents and therapists in learning about the consequences of brain injury and the special services that are needed to help the student continue his or her education.

- Specific educational processes and styles used in teaching head injury victims are very different from those used in teaching individuals who have permanent birth defects.

- Teachers may need to know the current medical issues and treatments your child is facing, your family dynamics, how you cope with crisis, some of your goals and wishes for your child, etc. You should also let the teachers know that you will advocate for your child but want to do so in a way that does not create problems for them.

- Working together and having compassion and respect for each other will help the process move more smoothly, but don't ever hesitate to speak up in a controlled manner and fight for your child.

- If your child is able, he or she can, with the proper plan in place, begin to reintegrate back into school. This can help spark brain waves into motion and reconnecting.

- Contact your local school board and ask to meet with the special needs coordinator.

- Contact the principal of your local school as soon as possible after injury. This will give the school time to prepare.

Going back to school, your child may or may not experience:

• Fear

• Irritability, angry outbursts, and impulsiveness

• Passive behavior

• Depression

• Confusion

• Forgetfulness

• A lack of organizational skills

• A hard time following directions

• Immature behavior

• Inappropriate sexual behavior

• Light and noise sensitivity

• Headaches

• Fatigue

• An inability to concentrate

• A lack of ability to retain information

• Long- or short-term memory loss

The Individual Education Plan (IEP)

• Each child needs his or her own IEP implemented according to his or her specific needs.

• Contact your school principal with your child's diagnosis of traumatic brain injury (have a physician put it in writing), and state that you wish to have an IEP developed and put into place.

• The IEP is a contract between the student, the parents, and the school. It will be the guide that helps your child succeed in the educational process and that helps you address your child's needs and accommodations.

• Every state has a law of education that must meet the federal requirements and may provide additional services.

• Set up a meeting with the school administrators to identify and discuss your child's abilities and difficulties. Bring background information from the rehabilitation hospital and a name of a physician or therapist who can help the school develop an appropriate program. To do this, you will need (at the cost of your school or insurance company or through the rehabilitation hospital) to obtain a neuropsychological evaluation for your child.

• Neurophysiologists have special training in relationships between brain function and behavior. They will evaluate your child to see how his or her injury affects learning, communication, planning, organization, and relationships with others. They can help develop an educational plan that best meets your child's needs. Through specific testing, a neurophysiologist can evaluate your child's cognitive abilities and deficits and provide teachers with suggestions and methods to stimulate and improve new learning. Neurophysiologists can also watch and identify changes as your child gets older.

• Think about your child's needs and look for services that best meet those needs.

• If your child is attending a rehabilitation outpatient program, the staff can work with the teachers by giving advice and helping create a program if your child will need occupational, speech, or physical therapy during school hours.

- Social workers can discuss resources with you and provide information about community support for the family, as well as provide adjustment counseling.

- Contact your state's brain injury association for added help and resources.

- Advocate for your child. Know your rights and those of your child under the law for education.

- If you are having communication problems or other issues with your school system, contact a professional educational advocate who can help you through the hurdles.

- Have a professional and knowledgeable person who knows about head injury meet with school administrators to explain the physical and cognitive changes that may be encountered.

- A rehabilitation therapist from your child's outpatient facility or someone from your current school system can help develop a behavior intervention plan.

- Ask school administrators to talk with and prepare the classmates for your child's return to school. It's helpful for peers to understand your child's limitations so that they can help, eg, carry books, give encouragement, sit with your child at lunch, etc.

- Start the transition back to school slowly—a few hours, two or three days a week, without educational demands. Increase attendance gradually as energy increases. Eventually your child may be able to attend full days, five days a week.

- Check on transportation options.

Think about the types of accommodations or assistance or types of assistive technology your child may need when transitioning back into school. Some ideas:

• Elevator availability and accessibility (if your child has difficulty with mobility)

• A personal aide to reinforce learning strategies

• Someone to help get lunch at the cafeteria

• Someone to help ambulate through the corridors

• A voice recording device

• Scheduled rest periods

• A transportation plan

• Remember that reintegrating into the social aspect of school is often just as vital as the academics, and that being included in school activities is important.

• Undergoing speech, occupational, and physical therapy during school hours will take up a lot of your child's academic time, and he or she may need any of the following: short tutoring sessions, computer access, books on tape, a scribe, additional time to complete tests, a lightened work load, a shortened day, etc.

• Know your child's schedule, and talk with teachers and therapists daily or weekly.

• Initiate meetings so you will have the opportunity to discuss teaching plans with everyone working with your child. Know what is working, and make a plan for what is not. If you tend to become too emotional, ask someone else who can advocate for your child to come with you and voice your concerns.

• Always thank and be kind to those who are trying to help, but do not be afraid to be assertive at times if needed.

• Set meeting dates for reviews, but do not hesitate to call the teachers any time.

• Long-range goals may change as your child's abilities become clearer.

• A child who has sustained a mild or moderate brain injury with no lasting physical disabilities can create a false sense of need, and other classmates or teachers may not realize these children have disabilities regarding memory loss, reasoning skills, concentration, behavioral issues, understanding subtle humor or directions, etc.

• Have one journal that is passed to each therapist and teacher during the day so that they can record and update the day's events and what was accomplished. Bring the journal home at the end of every day so you can read it and relay any questions or concerns.

• Your child may need a personal aide to accompany him or her throughout the school day. Make sure that your child and the aide get along well. If possible, the aide should have training in special education.

• Trust that you made the best decision for your child and family.

• Thank God for huge miracles.

• Ask people not to use the word "plateau." Realistically know your child's limitations, but continue to believe that he or she will keep going and going.

• On the first day of school, accompany your child and help the teachers and therapists get to know him or her. This also gives you an opportunity to see how they interact with your child.

• Use the time while your child is in school to deal with insurance companies, pay bills, get your house back in order, seek counseling, rest, or do nothing!

9

Going Forward

- As weeks turn into months and your life starts to settle down, even slightly, you may begin to have short bits of time when you start to realize all that you have been through and to see more clearly some of your child's lingering deficits. It is hard to accept that your child will never be the same person he or she was before traumatic brain injury. Brain injury does not go away. Acceptance comes with time and loving your child unconditionally.

- You may find that the sound of an ambulance or the sight of a hospital can bring you to tears. You may relive and experience flashbacks to the day of the injury. Your emotions may surface and be uncontrollable. It's all normal, but you could be experiencing post-traumatic stress disorder, which needs to be addressed by a physician.

- You may feel exhausted and have bouts of depression and a great feeling of loss. You may have body aches or severe headaches. Seek help.

- Try to escape for a weekend alone or with your partner or a friend. You may think there's no way that anyone is going to take care of your child or other children and your other responsibilities…but it is imperative that you find resources to help so that you have a reprieve. You need to take care of yourself!

- Feelings of grief and sadness may recur, even years later, and remind you of the horror and your lost hopes and dreams.

- Outpatient therapies may be starting to feel monotonous, but they are important to keep your child moving forward.

• You may begin to see your child's friends start to distance themselves. Call them or their parents and set times during the week when they could visit. The isolation that a head injury brings to its victims is heartbreaking. Do not force siblings to take the place of friends.

• Realize you have been through a catastrophic hardship and you, too, have to heal and come to terms with the aftermath. You too have been isolated in the emergency room, the trauma center, the ICU, the rehabilitation hospital, the outpatient therapies, and now at home. Be kind to yourself: allow yourself to start living again, go out to lunch, read a book, watch a movie, get a massage, get your hair done, or just take a walk along the beach...

• Caregiving is exhausting! Many caregivers have to readjust to their child's needs as the situation changes, including monitoring for behavior changes, cognitive strategies, safety issues, meal planning, medications, etc. Bathing, dressing, and personal care, structuring and planning activities and transporting to and from therapies...the list is endless. Although it's hard to ask for help, if you do not, you will burn out or worse.

• Teach others to do your job in case you are no longer able to do so or in case of an emergency. Give suggestions to those who want to help you— it is not a weakness to know your limits and to ask for help. Ultimately, it will help your child and give you more tolerance and energy.

• Try meditation, yoga, or another form of relaxation. Plan rest periods. Try to do at least one thing for yourself every day; otherwise you may become resentful.

• Seek out people who are in your situation and support and help one another.

• Include humor in your life; watch old sitcoms (eg, "I Love Lucy" reruns) or other silly shows.

• Local and state resources are available to help you and your child. Examples include the National Alliance for Caregiving, the National Family Caregivers Association, the National Respite Coalition, and the National Respite Locator Services.

- Remember no matter how bad your circumstances are, they always could be worse.

- Know that you and your family's collective caregiving and unconditional love makes all of you silent heroes. If your child was able to comprehend all that you have done and are still doing for him or her, you would receive a huge thank you at the end of every day!

Miracles Do Happen

- Bad stuff does happen, but you need to see the good parts of everything.

- Make the most of your lives and choices, but always remember to have a sense of humor.

- Be thankful for all that is in your life.

- Choose to react to your situation with a sense of faith, hope, patience, and a lot of love, humor, and passion.

- Through your experience, you have been startled from your slumber to awaken to a life that is fragile, a gift, and worth living…through the spectacular and the horrific…realizing more that each person is special, has meaning, a purpose.

- A higher power has been sustaining you, will continue to guide you, and is always there. Take time out of your busy day to listen and to pray.

- Perhaps the ultimate loss would be to lose our souls while still living, to give up on God, ourselves, our world.

- Those of us who have had a brush with death realize more deeply how fleeting life is. Make it great! Tell others often how much you love them and try to never take anyone for granted.

- Continue to help your child with perseverance and determination and by the grace of God.

- Celebrate life!

One Year Later

- To deal with the "new" person who emerges after brain injury, families must mourn the loss of the "old" one who is gone…and then move on to embrace life's challenges and changes and to love unconditionally.

- The fragility and meaning of life may become more real. Many families find new qualities, insights, and purpose to their days that would not have surfaced if the injury had not happened. Everyone can and will attest to the fact that they wished it had never happened.

- Hopefully, you will come to accept life's obstacles and adjust to the situation. At some point, you may even escape from your own cocoon and realize how your life has been transformed, to hopefully realize that you too can help others navigate through traumatic brain injury. To help one person, one family live through the **unthinkable**, giving a better understanding of new terrain…to reach out and give HOPE.

As Your Child gets Older

- The reality is…every brain injury and recovery and every family's experience with traumatic brain injury will be unique, depending on the specific circumstances and individual patient. **How you choose to react is the only thing that is in your power!**

- You will have to discern if your child is ready or capable of transitioning to college or to a vocational school or into the working world.

- You will need to consider whether your adult child will be able to live on his or her own, and if you need to investigate housing options that can provide assistance.

- You must also decide who will become your child's guardian and caregiver if you should become ill or die.

10

Siblings

The Forgotten Ones
How Parents Can Support Siblings

A collection of the tips specific for sibling-care

I

- At some point in life, everyone must face grief, suffering, and death.

- The only thing you can control is how you react to the events of life, including tragedies.

- It is impossible to completely shield your other children from emotional suffering. Do not feel guilty.

- All children fear the unknown. After a brain injury, the future is uncertain.

- TBI changes every member of a family. It is important to honor your children's views of the situation and the process by which they have coped (to whatever degree) with the staggering changes your family is experiencing.

- Appreciate that each child's situation, symptoms, and recovery are unique.

• Make sure to have someone you trust in charge of taking care of your other children when you're not home—and that it is someone your children like and can relate to.

• Check on your children often by phone, text messaging or e-mail. Reassure them and allow them to cry, vent, and show their fears. Try best to answer their questions, and when words cannot console…consider praying.

II

• Siblings may often feel isolated or resentful. They may perceive, no matter how hard parents try to not be so preoccupied with the ill/injured child, that they are rejected, unloved, or abandoned.

• Involve siblings from the beginning. Keep them informed of their brother's or sister's health condition in an age-appropriate manner. Talk one-on-one or give them written, audio, or video information through different phases of the injury or recovery.

• Conversations about the sibling's illness and or possible death or lingering deficits will need to be repeated as the child's understanding evolves.

• Let your healthy children know that their needs matter, too—and that they are just as important as their ill or injured sister or brother.

• Siblings often feel that it isn't okay to show or express how they truly feel, keeping their feelings bottled up inside.

• Encourage children to talk about their feelings, fears, and insecurities so you can better know how to help in a way unique for each child's needs. Let them know that feelings of guilt, shame, jealousy, grief, fear, resentment, abandonment, anger, anxiety, and denial are normal. Thoughts or feelings such as "why me?...why my family?...why my brother/sister?" are all normal.

• Be available to listen—not to try to fix the problem, but to validate your other children's feelings. "I hear how painful this is for you, or you sound scared. I am, too. We will be okay… together we can get through this…." Encourage children to talk about feelings as circumstances changes. Often kids think, "I have to be the strong one." "I don't want to cause mom or dad more pain."

III

- Tell your children how much you miss them when you have to leave. Let them know that you'll be back to give them updates on their brother or sister and that you will think of them while you're gone.

- You can never overuse the words "I LOVE YOU." Leave a note in lunch boxes or on pillows or the bathroom mirror.

- Include siblings in decision-making matters, such as how chores will be done, or devise a schedule for parent time with the healthy children or when siblings can visit their brother/sister.

- Let your older children know they are appreciated and thank them for helping with chores around the house or childcare. Enlist neighbors to help ease the burden of constant cooking, cleaning, yardwork, etc.

- Try to stick to the child's schedule as much as possible, including regularly attending both school and after-school activities.

- Help children understand why and how the injury happened. Younger children often blame themselves, while older children may question if they could have prevented the injury; reassure them there was nothing they could have done.

- Give reassurance that the injured child is getting good care and that you're doing everything possible to help their brother/sister.

- Encourage your other children to write cards or send pictures to help decorate the hospital room.

- When it's time to bring your other children to the hospital, talk to the hospital's child life department, which helps siblings and grandparents cope with the situation and prepare for the visit.

• Trying to take care of your other children's emotions when they visit the hospital can be challenging. Try to have a nurse, friend, or your spouse/partner with you.

• Never force your other children to visit; wait for them to ask. Help prepare children by giving them age-appropriate written and verbal information on brain injury. Give them time to absorb the information and the situation.

• Identify "time-out areas" for siblings during the hospital visit. Possibilities include the playroom, a "family" room, lounge, cafeteria.

• Be truthful. Explain what the doctors are doing and hope to accomplish, but also let children (in age-appropriate terms) and grandparents know the reality of life and possible death.

IV

• Grief often comes in waves.

• Remember that grief is a natural response to loss; it does not need to have to be a way of life.

• Seek help through the school or hospital's counseling department.

• It's normal for siblings to have conflict; they may resist going to school or studying, or act out. Let teachers know what happened, and seek out school counselors to help with the new terrain. Some kids may need tutors or extra time to complete school work or be given a lightened load.

• Hold onto hope and give an abundance of hugs.

• Have your other children seek out positive people to be around: counselors, clergy, friends, a special nurse or teacher.

• Your children may be suffering other losses: familiar routines, sense of identity and security, feeling of being in control of life situations, care-free days, and the normalcy of everyday life.

• If siblings have become "quiet," do not assume that they are okay or have accepted the situation; often, they do not want to add to your burden.

• If a child's mood or behavior becomes extreme (sadness, excessive talk of death or dying, violent outbursts of anger), it may be necessary to seek professional help.

• Pay attention to changes in behavior and sleep patterns. Depending on the signs and symptoms, your other children may need psychiatric evaluations, sleep aids, or antidepressants.

• Realize life goes on for your children's friends, while your children are trying to adjust to their new situation. Siblings often feel isolated from their peers.

• Keep an eye on the older children for possible alcohol consumption or the use of drugs to escape their new reality.

V

• As hard as it is, try to take time away from the hospital to give attention to your other children.

• Meet as a family to find out how everyone is coping.

• When you are home, find time to talk to each child alone and on his or her level. For example, take one child with you while you run errands, or for a special ice cream treat and talk.

• Keep communication open and going with all your children. When you're able, try to spend 15-30 minutes a day alone with each child. Turn off the computer, the television, the I-pods. Give your children your undivided attention. A good way to keep communicating (especially with a child who tends to be quieter) is for each child to have a diary that is intended for you to share only with each other. Sometimes, a diary allows kids to better express themselves or to ask questions in a way that is "safe." You can write back and forth to clarify, reassure, and answer difficult questions. Drawing also helps some children to explain or share their thoughts and feelings.

• Help your children be educated on TBI and the recovery process.

• Give daily updates to your other children on their sibling's recovery, however incremental.

• Know that your moods and those of your other children will change daily when critical moments and difficult situations arise.

• Let siblings know that counseling and support systems are there when they are ready.

• Communicate the possible realities of permanent loss of memory, mobility, hearing, sight, speech…

• Ask children what they understand about the situation, and allow children to ask questions. Answer the questions as honestly as possible. Children are very perceptive and know when parents are trying to hide something from them.

• It is okay to cry with your children, but try to keep them anchored and hopeful whenever possible.

• If your other children want to be involved with their sibling's therapies, make every attempt to include them.

• Help your children to realize that recovery may be lifelong.

• Help your other children understand and accept the possibility that the person they once new may never be returned to them.

• Give an abundance of hugs!

• Celebrate milestones: first time speaking, moving a finger, making eye contact…

• Remember that small gains are big miracles.

VI

• Children often feel isolated from their peers, feeling like no one understands what they are going through. Offer Web sites for older siblings, picture books for younger children, or other resources your children can use to relate to other TBI siblings.

• Give siblings their space when needed, but leave time for them to be together so they can vent and cry and share. Let them know it is okay to let down their guard and to cry, kick, or scream.

• Communicate frequently with teachers of siblings to make sure you are aware of any developing problems.

• People constantly asking your children about the welfare of the injured child can be overwhelming. Give them a standard sentence to reply with such as, "Thank you for asking. My brother/sister is stable, and we are taking it one day at a time."

• Don't worry too much about how other extended family members are coping. Concentrate on your child, yourself, your other children, and your spouse/partner.

• Realize you are not alone; other people before you have experienced your sorrow and have come through the tunnel.

• Take care of yourself. Rest when you can and eat properly so you can have the energy and ability to take care of your other children.

• Keep communication going between you and your spouse/partner to help advocate for each other and your other children.

• Try to keep extracurricular actives going for your other children as much as possible. Ask neighbors and friends to help with schedules and rides and to help with childcare and food preparations to lessen the burden on older siblings.

• Although the holidays will never be like they used to, try to make them as normal as possible by keeping with your traditions. Ask a friend to shop and decorate for you.

VII

• If your injured child is able to return home, prepare your other children for the transition. Start talking with doctors and counselors. Take advantage of your safety net while you can, because soon you will be on your own.

• Some children may think their brother or sister is cured when it's time to return home. Let them know injuries still linger and what they are: cognitive, physical…

• Try to prepare your other kids for more changes ahead. They may feel embarrassed by the behaviors of the injured child and may avoid being home or inviting friends over.

• Others in your community may think that just because you are home you no longer need help. Communicate that you are still in need of help! Cooking, cleaning, childcare, carpools…and comfort.

• Keep advocating for the needs of your family. If you can afford it, hire a housekeeper, nanny, marriage counselor, etc, if needed.

• Know that a lot of emotions will surface once your child is home. Be prepared for reactions from your injured child as well as from your other children. They will be apprehensive and unsure as to how life could ever be the same. Be reassuring—you all will slowly adjust to the changes with time and with help from each other.

• If one child is demanding more attention and you're unable to be there, enlist extended family and friends to help.

• Social workers can discuss resources with you and provide information about community support for the family, as well as provide adjustment counseling.

- Perhaps your children may benefit from joining a support group for siblings who have a brother or sister with TBI.

- Memory issues are a huge problem for victims of TBI, and they affect the whole family. Using a white-board and calendar can help if your child is able to read. Reinforce the day's schedule, what activities were accomplished, what is happening, etc.

- Your family will go through many adjustments. Don't give up! Adjusting to a new way of life and trying to find some sort of a "new" normalcy takes some trial and error.

- Suggest ways in which your other children can help, or give them time to back off. Do not force siblings to take the place of the injured child's friends.

VIII

- Remember that how you react to any given situation is in your power.

- Your other children will have to adjust to other's reactions when they see their injured sibling in public. Let them know to smile, be polite, and to say a prayer for others that they will never have to be in this situation.

- Be thankful that your family is all together under one roof.

- As weeks turn into months and sometimes years, and your life starts to settle down, even slightly, you may begin to have short bits of time when you start to realize all that you have been through and to see more clearly some of your child's lingering deficits. It may be hard for you and your other children to accept that your child may never be the same person he or she was before TBI. Brain injury does not go away. Acceptance comes with time and unconditional love.

- The fragility and meaning of life may become more real. Many families find new qualities, insights, and purpose to their days that would not have surfaced if the injury had not happened. Everyone can and will attest to the fact that they wished it had never happened.

• Life must and should move forward for your other children, but they can take lessons learned from TBI as they go out into the world.

• Those of us who have come near to death realize more deeply how fleeting life is. Make it great! Tell others often how much you love them, and try never to take your children or anyone for granted.

Celebrate life!

• Hopefully, your children will come to accept life's unforeseen obstacles and adjust to the situation with help and your continued love. At some point, they may even escape from their heartache and realize that they, too, can help others navigate through TBI. To help one person, one family live through the **unthinkable,** giving a better understanding of the new terrain…to reach out and give HOPE.

• Years have now passed since my son's crash when he sustained a severe TBI, which changed every member of our family. Many people still ask how we did it…how did our family survive and triumph through such tragedy? I always answer, "We never gave up… on God, ourselves, our world."

Afterword

TBI Ten Years Later: A Mother's Story Continues

It has been almost ten years since traumatic brain injury (TBI) crashed into our lives, changing our family forever. People always ask, "How is your son Paul doing now? How are you, your husband, the other kids? How has your family survived?" I usually give my polite, standard answer: "Oh…thanks for asking, we're all doing fine. And you?" But the reality is—unless you have experienced the loss, the heartache, and the ripple effects that brain injury can inflict—you cannot possibly understand the magnitude and the seriousness of the life-altering implications. The long-term impact that TBI imposes on the injured person, family members, and friends is unthinkable. The nightmare of TBI relives itself day after day, month after month, and year after year. Grief and sadness persist even ten years later, despite all the miraculous gains my son has made since his initial injury.

After the shock of Paul's accident and TBI diagnosis when I understood the reality and severity of his injuries, knowing that they were likely to include lingering deficits and handicaps   I wanted to bury my head under a pillow and slip under a thick blanket of denial. But to survive, I realized the necessity of being strong-willed and maintaining an attitude of never giving up. Everyone—myself and my family as well as the doctors, nurses, therapists, and even Paul himself—would have to draw on inner resources we had not known existed.

In the early stages of Paul's injury, he was immobile and essentially in a vegetative state. We suddenly had to become his eyes, his ears, his voice. We needed to advocate for his every need. My husband and I fought to find the best medical, financial, educational, legal, vocational, and rehabilitation services available. We never stopped advocating for our son's needs or for those of our family. As days turned into months, and months turned into years, I do not know where our energy or drive came from to venture into areas we knew nothing about. But there was no way we would stand idle without trying to help our son possibly regain even some of what he had lost after being struck by a car while riding his bike at age 13.

We came to realize that the outcome of each TBI, like each person, is unique. A person's outcome depends on the specific circumstances and severity of the injury, immediate and long-term medical care, rehabilitation services, and the individual patient and family. We also learned that many people with TBI plateau relatively soon after their injury, without making huge gains. Sometimes these injured people and their families are left to cope with so much beyond their control: cognitive, memory, behavioral, physical, emotional, and social changes...the medical bills and never-ending insurance claims...the everyday demands of cooking, laundry, cleaning, yard work, going to the office, maintaining a marriage, and keeping other children's studies and activities moving forward.

Rehabilitation: After many months in ICU, our son was stabilized, but the urgency continued. Getting him into a rehabilitation hospital was key to learning how to speak, to walk, and to perform basic tasks again. We knew Paul's recovery was questionable and that he could possibly remain bedridden, wheelchair-bound, or cognitively impaired. But the months of grueling shifts of speech, occupational, and physical therapies began to pay off. Paul fought back like a champion! We began to see small gains—he blinked his eyelids, lifted a finger, uttered a word. Seeing the healing begin was powerful and moving. Yet Paul still had a long way to go.

Reintegrating Home: Anticipating Paul's release from the rehabilitation hospital, we were faced with a new set of questions. What would we do next? Paul was still using a wheelchair and a walker. He was still struggling with memory and speech loss. He still needed assistance with everyday activities and self-care. I worried about how we were going to cope. When my husband or I were home, we'd tried to focus on the needs and cares of our other children, while managing the daily chores that made the household run smoothly. When we'd been at the rehab hospital, our only focus had been to take care of Paul. I was not sure how, or if, it would even be possible, to mesh these two demanding worlds into one.

I knew our family would be under more stress and would have to surpass the extraordinary level of support and help we were already extending to each another. We had to think about all aspects of home nursing and medical care, to obtain and install all assistive and adaptive equipment, and to prepare Paul's siblings for the homecoming of their "new" brother. We suggested ways for the other kids to help, and we gave them permission to back off if need be. The caregiving was both never ending and exhausting. We had to recognize our own limitations, shed any guilt, and ask for help from our community, friends, and family.

Outpatient Therapy: Continuing outpatient therapies was important to help Paul regain more movement and thinking capabilities. We logged many miles driving to and from his new outpatient facility, 20 minutes from home. I was shocked at how many injured or maimed people came and went every half hour. Missing legs and arms could have been one of the criteria for entry. And the therapies went on and on and on....

Reintegrating Back to School: We tried relentlessly to set up home tutoring through our town's special education department to get Paul the mental stimulation he needed to continue recovery. But after investigating special needs schools and other facilities, we made the hard choice to try to reintegrate Paul into the public school system. We recognized the challenge because specific educational processes and styles used in teaching TBI students are very different from those used in teaching individuals who have permanent birth defects. Paul needed an Individual Educational Plan (IEP) geared toward his specific needs. He underwent a neurophysiology examination, which is concerned with the relationships between brain function and behavior and considers how injury may affect learning, communication, planning, organization, and relationships with others. The neurophysiologist evaluated Paul's cognitive abilities and deficits and provided teachers with suggestions and methods to stimulate and improve new learning. In other words, the evaluation was used to help develop Paul's IEP. When Paul returned to school, the break from constant rehabilitation allowed our days to regain some degree of normalcy.

Friends and Family Relationships: All of our lives had changed dramatically since Paul's accident. I know Paul felt the absence of the phone not ringing, and of his friends no longer coming by to hang out. With the time that had passed, most of his friends had distanced themselves. Some were just typical self-centered teenagers, but others could not relate to the slowness with which Paul now talked and walked, and could not comprehend the differences, though slight, in Paul's personality. To his peers, Paul appeared childlike, odd, and different. To adults, Paul was an inspiration of hope. His subtle humor made everyone smile.

Over time, my husband and I and our other seven children began to realize two things: the person we once knew might never be returned to us, and recovery would be lifelong. Because all of our lives had been put on hold for so long while we coped with such staggering changes, we started to nurture all of our family relationships. We gave permission to each other to start moving forward, to begin to go back to our daily routines, including even recreational activities.

Getting a Job: As time went on, Paul's mobility and his physical, mental, and cognitive abilities improved. He no longer needed the special school accommodations that we had fought for so desperately: the personal aide, the small classroom atmosphere, a personal computer, scheduled rest periods, books on tape, and so forth. At Paul's high school graduation, he walked to the podium to receive his diploma—no wheelchair, no walker but a clear understanding of all that he had accomplished. But leaving school also meant leaving the only support system we knew. The fight would continue, and we would have to again advocate for Paul to help him find employment and become more independent. Working with our state's rehabilitation office, Paul gained employment at a local retail store where he started as a greeter, quickly moving up to sales clerk and then cashier.

Higher Education: Paul is not the same person he was before the crash. He walks off-balance, though to his family, it is a blessing he walks at all. His voice is slow and monotone. Yet, we are extremely grateful that he can speak. Cognitively, he may be slightly slower to process information, to form a thought, or to respond to a question. But the reality of his ability to react with maturity, humor, and intelligence is beyond our belief. The tremors and shakes that affect the left side of his body make it hard for him to do almost everything. But his persistence and perseverance are mind-boggling. Ten years after Paul sustained a TBI, he volunteered at the hospital where his life was saved. He speaks at rehab hospitals, medical facilities, and preventive organizations talking about TBI and the importance of wearing a bike helmet. Remarkably, he is in a higher education program, attending Lesley University (The Threshold Program) in Boston, where he is living independently, surrounded by other young adults.

Ten Years Later: Despite all the miraculous gains my son has made over the years, my heart often remains heavy. When I look into my husband's or my children's eyes, I can still see the lingering fear, the permanent scars.

To deal with the "new" person who emerges after brain injury, families must mourn the loss of the "old" one who is gone…and then move on to embrace life's challenges and changes and to love unconditionally. The fragility and meaning of life have indeed become more real as my family has found new qualities, insights, and purpose to our days that would not have surfaced if the injury had not happened. And even ten years later, the sound of an ambulance or the sight of a hospital can evoke tears as we relive and experience flashbacks to that unthinkable day of the accident.

Ten years later, my heart also remains heavy as I think of other families who will receive the unthinkable news that one of their loved ones has sustained a life-altering injury. I understand all too well the grief and uphill battles they are sure to encounter. I also pray that these families will reach out to get help and resources, to have the strength and will to advocate, to never give up…and to keep hope alive.

TBI Resources

National Family Caregivers Association
http://www.nfcacares.org/

National Rehabilitation Information Center
http://naric.com/

National Association of State Head Injury Administrators
http://www.nashia.org/

National Institute of Neurological Disorders and Stroke
http://www.ninds.nih.gov/about_ninds/addresses.htm

International Brain Injury Association
http://www.internationalbrain.org/

Brain Injury Association of America
http://www.biausa.org/

American Brain Tumor Association
http://www.abta.org/

North American Brain Injury Society
http://www.nabis.org/

Brain Injury of Canada
http://www.biac-aclc.ca/

Defense and Veterans Brain Injury Center
http://www.dvbic.org/

Brainline.org
http://www.brainline.org/index.html

Lash and Associates Publishing/Training Inc.
http://www.lapublishing.com/blog/lash-associates-publishing/

Mothers Against Brain Injury, Inc.
http://www.mabii.org/

Unthinkable: A Mother's Tragedy, Terror, and Triumph through a Childs's Traumatic Brain Injury
www.dixiecoskie.com

Motherhood

I had always wanted to be an astronaut to see if there were galaxies beyond our planet, to venture to where eternity began or infinity ended.

I had always dreamed of being an architect to create and bring to life an outrageous house sitting on a cliff singing to the ocean.

I had always thought to travel to explore the Greek gods, to play in the pyramids, and to climb the highest peaks in the land.

Never in my wildest dreams could I have imagined that motherhood could be so mystical, adventurous, rewarding, challenging, fulfilling, and so grand.

~ Dixie

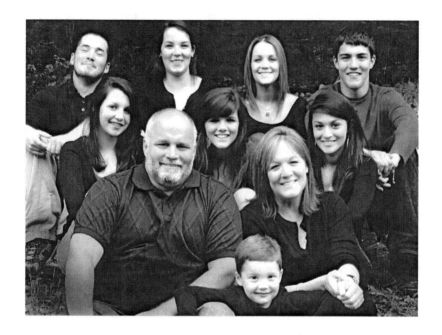

2009 Coskie Family Picture:
Jack (in front)
next row – Steven (Dad), Dixie (Mom)
second row left to right – Monica, Anna-Theresa, Caroline
third row – Paul, Amanda, Brianna, Kevin

Courtesy of William Lukas Photography Center

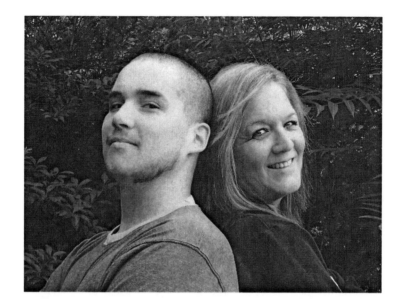

Contact the Author

Dixie Coskie and her son Paul speak at schools, camps, trauma centers, hospitals and rehab hospitals talking about the consequences and the reality of traumatic brain injury, and also on childhood cancer.

Contact Dixie for booking information
email: dixie@dixiecoskie.com or call 508-320-0425

Please feel free to contact us
for media interviews
to have Dixie or Paul Coskie speak at your next event
to contribute to your next book club
If you have a question or need more information
or to share thoughts about *Unthinkable* or your own story

Notes